30 Day Kettlebell WOD Exercises!

I0417120

Kettlebell

Get In Shape Fast With Amazing Russian Kettlebell And Cross Training Workouts!

Chris Smith

STOP!!! Before you read any further....Would you like to know the Secrets of Body Transformation?

If your answer is yes, then you are not alone. Thousands of people are looking for the secret to rapidly burn body fat, keep the weight off, become healthier, and truly transform their body and life for good.

If you have been searching for these answers without much luck, you are in the right place!

Not only will you gain incredible insight in this book, but because I want to make sure to give you as much value as possible, right now for a limited time you can get full **100% FREE access to a VIP bonus EBook** entitled **THE 7 KEYS TO BODY TRANSFORMATION!**

Legal Notice

Disclaimer Notice

Table Of Contents

Introduction

I want to thank you and congratulate you for purchasing the book, *30 Day Kettlebell WOD Exercises!*

This "Kettlebell" book contains proven steps and strategies on how to lose weight and tone your muscles using only the Russian kettlebell.

This book covers all the factors that affect weight loss including workouts, resting and diet. By using the tips suggested in this book, you will be able to lose weight fast without the need for expensive equipment. The kettlebell exercises are really easy and they could also be integrated to the workouts that you are already doing. The nutrition principle suggested by this book follows the Paleo and low carb diet. We hope that you will reach your workout goals by using the tips suggested in this book.

Thanks again for purchasing this book, I hope you enjoy it!

Chapter 1: Workout Principles

There are no shortcuts to losing weight. You have to do your part to be able to achieve your dream body. The amount of work needed will vary depending on your current fitness status and your fitness goals.

Set your Goals

Every important achievement starts with a goal. It will be easier to accomplish your fitness achievement if you also start it with a goal. In stating our goals, we need to make sure that they are specific. It should not be open to any other interpretation. If you aim to lose weight, you should have a number of kilograms or pounds stated in your goal. If it is about having abs, you should measure the diameter of your tummy and you should look for a picture of a fit and toned abs to use as reference.

Your goal should also have a deadline, but make sure that it is realistic. Ensure that you can accomplish your goals according to the deadline that you set. Setting a deadline that is too near will leave you frustrated because you will not be able to reach your goals on time. Setting a deadline that is too far may also lead you to fail. People usually procrastinate when they have too much time to finish a goal.

Lastly, your fitness goals should be reachable based on your resources. You should make sure that you have access to all the things that you need to reach your goals.

People who start working out usually have two common goals in mind; to lose weight and to look good. You should stop and think after this chapter to assess what you want to achieve in getting into the kettlebell WOD program suggested by this book. You should put it into writing and paste it in a place where you will always see it.

Your additional goal:

Aside from your personal goals, it is the duty of every workout mentor to encourage you to keep a healthy lifestyle. After reaching the goals that you set today, you must set more goals to work for.

If you continue to do this, you will be able to make your workouts a part of your lifestyle. By doing this, the fitness accomplishments that you achieve will become permanent. You will have a toned physique and an athletic frame even when you grow older. You will also be able to maintain a healthy weight even as you enter middle age. This is usually the time when people start failing to meet their scheduled workouts and start gaining weight and beer belly.

The Role of Nutrition

Though this book focuses on the workouts, it also teaches the role of nutrition in your weight loss and fitness goals. Just because you workout often doesn't mean that you can eat any type or amount of food that you like. We will discuss the best kind of diet that will best work with your high intensity workouts.

This will be discussed in the later parts of the book.

Chapter 2: Using The Russian Kettlebell To Get In Shape

The kettlebell, which originated from Russia, is one of the most effective exercise tools to have in your home or office. Many workout gurus claim that you can achieve all of your fitness goals using this simple and cheap workout tool. This book doesn't just claim that; we will also teach you how to do it.

Before we go to the specific workout moves that you can do, let us first discuss why you should choose using the kettlebell instead of the other workout contraptions that you see in TV ads.

It's cheap

One of the most basic sources of appeal for the kettlebell is its low price. The kettlebell that you have today will last for the rest of your life. Unlike the workout machines that you find in gyms, it will not break or malfunction. Good quality kettlebells also don't rust. That means that they will be in good condition even when you've dripped sweat on them for a decade.

It's convenient to use and store

Unlike dumbbells and barbells, you don't have to change the weights in your kettlebell every time you change your exercise move. Each kettlebell has a specific weight. This means that you can immediately pick them up on your workout schedules and start pumping iron. Because you no longer have to deal with iron plates, you will have an easier time putting them away after each workout.

It can be used to work out your whole body

Many people think that kettlebells are the same as ordinary dumbbells. As you explore more of this book however, you will realize that the moves that you can do with kettlebells are a lot more diverse compared to dumbbells. You will be able to use kettlebells not only in strength training but also in improving your cardio-respiratory fitness. The exercises that use kettlebells also make use of more muscle groups compared to the common workout moves performed with barbells. The latter is mostly used in isolating muscle groups. With kettlebells, you have the choice to isolate one muscle group or work on multiple muscle groups simultaneously.

Its ergonomic design mimics carrying everyday objects

We normally carry the kettle ball in the same way we carry plastics of groceries or a briefcase. The wrist position and the suspended arms used when carrying kettle actually allows us to work on the same muscle movements that we execute everyday when we are doing everyday tasks. Using kettlebell will make us stronger in our everyday tasks. This is the reason why both men and women should start using kettlebells in their daily workout routines.

Chapter 3: The Kettlebell And CrossFit Training

Because of the versatility of kettlebells to be included in the training regimen of any athlete, it is constantly used in the workout regimen of CrossFit practitioners. The practitioners who use this tool in their CrossFit programs are usually focused in improving strength and power.

If you are not familiar with CrossFit, it is a popular strength and conditioning program used in gyms all around the world. The program aims to improve your overall fitness through a series of high-intensity workouts. The three main types of workouts that you will do in CrossFit are aerobics, gymnastics and Olympic weight lifting exercises. The exercises that you do will vary each day. Some CrossFit gyms also design programs for practitioners with specific physical needs like sports training, martial arts training or professional fitness.

A typical CrossFit workout session will include a series of warm up exercises followed by skill development workout. Then, the Workout of the Day or the WoD will follow. Each individual gym has their own prescribed workout of the day but there are also some who follow the workout of the day suggested by the CrossFit website. The session usually ends with stretching exercises to cool down them muscles. There are some gyms who concentrate their WoDs on improving the strength like using Olympic weight lifting.

After the session, your performance in executing the workout of the day will be scored and ranked compared to other people that you worked out with. Other people also time their workouts. This practice makes the gym atmosphere even more competitive.

Using Kettlebells

For fitness buffs who have limited workout equipment at home, using the prescribed workout of the day will not be successful in yielding results because of the necessary tools to do certain tasks. This is where the kettlebell will come in handy. Instead of following the WoD in the CrossFit website or the local gym, you could start practicing CrossFit in your own home just by using kettlebells. You could do this by using the kettlebell workouts of the day found in this book.

This method is cheaper than joining a gym. It is also a lot more feasible than following the prescribed workout of the day in the CrossFit website. It is also a good option for beginners who are not yet confident about their ability to complete one CrossFit session.

Using the 30-day cycle

In the next chapter, you will see a 30-day routine using only kettlebells. A month long practice of these suggested workouts will help build enough muscles and stamina to prepare you for even more CrossFit trainings.

It is also better if you try to work out with a friend or a family member. Aside from the high-intensity workouts, CrossFit's success is greatly due to the community behind it. Make sure that you become a member of local CrossFit communities in your area. You could find some of them in local sports clubs and gyms. The community not only increases your sense of competition but can also be a good source of information and tips to become better.

Chapter 4: 30 Day Kettlebell WOD Exercises

The key to completing the 30-day kettlebell challenge is balance. You need to achieve balance in your nutrition, workout schedule and resting time. This will prevent your body from not having enough energy or from becoming injured due to over fatigue.

For beginners, it may be necessary to limit the number of workout sessions per week to three. This is to ensure that your body will have time to recover from the grueling workout. If you are already fit, you can increase frequency of sessions per week to 5. You can set one workout session a day to suit your schedule.

If you are confident that you can finish the prescribed workouts in the table below, you could try to complete it. The 30-day routine suggested below only has one rest day every 7 days. This will yield faster weight loss results. Rest is also an essential part of losing weight. Make sure that you have at least 24 hours to rest before the next workout.

The warm ups

Before each session, you should warm up the muscles that you will use first. Because we are always using the muscles in the lower and upper arms, you need to stretch them out and condition them by lifting light weight kettlebells.

Here are some warm up moves that you do to prepare your muscles for the workout ahead:

Name of Exercise	Target Muscles
Shoulder strangle	Shoulder muscles
Hand Down Spine	Shoulders and Triceps
Forearm Rotation	Elbow and lower arms
Arm Rotation	Shoulders
Standing Quadriceps Stretch	Quadriceps

| Bar Twist | Hips |
| Side lunge | Leg muscles |

These are only some of the stretching exercises that you can use. You should choose the exercises that will stretch or warm up the muscle groups that you will use for the day.

The 30-day Workout of the Day Exercises

Day #	Kettlebell Exercise to Use	Target Muscle
1	Kettlebell Swing	Back, Shoulders, Hips, Gluteus, Legs
2	Kettlebell Power Plank with Row	Abdominal Muscles, Arms, Back
3	Kettlebell Goblet Squat	Back, Legs, Gluteus Muscles
4	Single Arm Kettlebell Floor Press	Arms, Chest, Core
5	Rest Day	
6	Kettlebell High Pull	Shoulders, Arms, Gluteus Muscles, Legs
7	Kettlebell Lunge Press	Back, Shoulders, Arms, Abdominal Muscles, Gluteus Muscles, Legs
8	Kettlebell Sumo High Pull	Back, Legs, Arms, Shoulders
9	Kettlebell Russian Twist	Abdominal Muscles, Lower Back
10	Kettlebell Windmill	Back, Shoulders, Abdominal Muscles, Oblique Muscles, hips

11	Extended Range One-arm Kettlebell Floor Press	Chest, Shoulder, Triceps
12	Rest Day	
13	Side step Kettlebell Swing	Legs, Gluteus Muscles, back
14	Kettlebell Pushup	Triceps, Chest
15	Single Arm Kettlebell Swing	Back, Shoulders, Hips, Gluteus, Legs
16	Kettlebell one-legged dead lift	Hamstrings, Gluteus Muscles, Lower Back
17	Kettlebell Pistol Squat	Quadriceps, Calves, Gluteus Muscles, Hamstrings, Shoulders
18	Leg Over Floor Press	Chest, Shoulders, Triceps
19	Rest Day	
20	Plyo Kettlebell Pushups	Chest, Shoulders, Triceps
21	Kettlebell Alternating Renegade Row	Back, Arms, Shoulders, Core, Hips, Legs
22	Front Squats with two Kettlebells	Quadriceps and Gluteus Muscles
23	Kettlebell Pushup with Row	Back, Chest, Arms
24	Kettlebell Half Get up	Abdominal Muscles, Arms, Back
25	Kettlebell Figure 8	Arms, Back, Abdominal Muscles
26	Rest Day	
27	Single Arm Kettlebell Split Jerk	Back, Shoulders, Chest, Legs

28	Two-Arm Kettlebell Military Press	Back, Shoulders, Arms
29	Kettlebell clean	Butt, Legs, Back
30	Kettlebell Dead lift	Legs, Gluteus Muscles, arms, back, Abdominal Muscles

When doing the workouts above, you should do 8-10 reps using a 16kg kettlebell for men. If 16 kg is too difficult for some movements like get-ups and windmills, use a 12 kg kettlebell. Gradually work your way up the weight ladder when 10 reps is too easy for you.

Beginner women should start with 6 to 10-kilogram kettlebell. They should also start with 8 reps. Instead of increasing weights however; women who only want to lose weight should increase the number of reps.

Incorporating the Kettlebell WOD to your CrossFit Routine

After doing 8-10 reps of the Kettlebell WOD, you should follow it with 10 pushups. You should try to finish the round as fast as you can. You should do 5 rounds of this workout pair during your workout days. You could have a minute to rest in between set. You could also change the pushups to other calisthenics exercises.

To make it more challenging, you could do the same exercises on the following month. However, this time, you will record the time that you used to finish the prescribed 5 rounds. You should do the same workout on the following month while trying to lessen the time to finish the routine.

Chapter 5: Cross Training

Aside from using kettlebells with the CrossFit program, you could also use it while practicing and preparing for another sport. CrossFit is often used by professionals who rely on their fitness to do their jobs properly. Many firemen, policemen and paramedics use it all over the country. You will benefit even more from this program if you join the sports that the CrossFit community around you plays.

By using cross training in your workout routines, you will expose your body to more movements that challenge every part of it. Focusing on only a few muscle groups all the time is inadequate if you want to develop overall fitness. People often feel out of shape when they are doing a new set of exercises or a new type of sports. A fitness buff who is used to working out his upper body may feel really out of shape when they are jogging. If you put a body builder in a running game like basketball, they often feel inadequate because of the lack of practice. They are not accustomed to the speed and the flexibility that the sport requires.

This is where cross training can help. By constantly looking for new sports and workout regimens to try, we are developing all the aspects of our fitness. We are also increasing our skill set not only in sports but also in the physical requirements of life.

How to start cross training

Train for two types of sports

You can handpick the workout moves suggested in this book to train for a sport. When studying a new sport, take note of the key movements that you need to practice and the muscles that you need to develop to be able to execute those movements effectively. You should then choose the kettlebell workouts of the day that target these movements.

Include flexibility and speed in your training

When cross training, you should never neglect the other aspects of fitness that most muscle-builders forget; flexibility and speed.

Luckily, the workouts that improve these aspects of fitness can be done with minimal equipment.

Learn a new sport every year

Many people only focus on two or three types of sports or workout activities when they are cross train. Some of them however, get tired of the monotony of these sports. The monotony in training also adds to the rigidity of the joints decreasing flexibility and agility. To keep your body in shape and to keep challenging it, you should learn a new sport ever year. Some people who have mastered sport swimming for example, transfer to learning surfing or diving. Choose sports that are related to the current sports that you are practicing.

Chapter 6: High Intensity Interval Training

Because we are following CrossFit principles in our training regimen, we must learn how to execute the High Intensity Interval Training properly. A typical CrossFit session lasts from 30 minutes to 1 hour. You can achieve results even with just a small duration of workout each day because of the use of HIIT.

As the name suggests this type of training uses the interval training method where in workout moves that release strong bursts of energy is followed by a very short period of rest before going to another high intensity workout move.

Using the HIIT, you can choose to focus on one muscle group for the day or to target multiple muscle groups. Your choice should depend in your goals. People who want to build muscles target one muscle group on each workout day to maximize muscle hypertrophy. The HIIT will work their muscles out to the point of exhaustion. After working it out, the muscle group will be allowed to rest for 2 days to allow the muscles to load itself up with protein. This will result to muscle growth and toning.

If you want a slender and toned body on the other hand, you should target multiple body parts on each workout day. This will lessen the chances of injury caused by repetitive use of a muscle. This type of HIIT will also increase your metabolic rate better compared to isolating one muscle group for each workout session.

How to start using HIIT

As with starting any new workout on your own, you should approach HIIT slowly as a beginner. The high intensity workouts are designed to boost the workout performance of athletes. If you are not confident with your athleticism yet, you could start out with short durations of high intensity exercises with resting time double or triple the sprint time.

20 seconds/60 seconds interval

You could start with these durations. The 20 seconds refer to the duration of your high intensity workout and 60 seconds refer to the duration of the resting state that follows.

For example, you could start by doing as many kettlebell snatches for 20 seconds. After that, you should rest for a minute. You should move on to the next workout move for another 20/60 seconds interval.

Chapter 7: Making Your Metabolism Work For You

Your weight loss goals are largely dependent on your metabolic rate. When working out to lose weight, you should not focus on the amount of calories you lose per workout. Instead, focus on increasing your metabolic rate every day. By doing this, you will maximize the effect of your workout by burning calories all throughout the day.

People who live a sedentary lifestyle have a difficult time losing weight because they spend most of their time in a rested state. When we rest, our body tries to conserve energy by making our metabolism slower. It is at its slowest when we are asleep.

Increasing your metabolism

Every time you work out, your body not only spends energy to do your reps and laps but it also spends it to repair your body afterwards. The repair and maintenance process that our body enters after a workout increases our metabolic rate. Your metabolism is the overall chemical processes that your body performs for its maintenance. The amount of chemical reactions that happen in your body is momentarily increased after your workouts to repair the body and to make it stronger the next time around. This increased metabolic rate means that your body is spending energy even though we are no longer working out.

For people who want to grow bigger muscles, it is essential to rest immediately after working out. The rest period allows our body to focus its attention on repair and maintenance. After it is done with what it needs to do, the body gradually returns to a normal metabolic rate.

If you want to lose weight, you must prolong the periods of high metabolic rate. This period shortens if you rest or sleep after your workouts. If you remain awake and active after a high-intensity workout however, you can prolong this period.

To maximize the effects of your workout routines, you should schedule your workouts in the morning before you go to the office. The high intensity workouts suggested in this book will speed up your metabolism early in the morning. This increased metabolic rate will continue even as you go to work. Your heart rate will be faster than usual. You will be spending more energy in your office time until your body has done all the repairs and maintenance that it needs to do.

Some people who aren't used to working out in the morning become easily winded out when they start this habit. Over time however, you will be used to the feeling and you will be able to work through it.

Chapter 8: How Weight Loss Happens

The number of days where you increase your metabolism is also important. It should be done often and regularly for you to consistently lose weight. You will be able to reach your target weight fast if you create a habit of working out using the kettlebell system and eating the right types and amounts of food.

During your workouts, your body will try to provide you with energy in lifting by using up the glucose, a simple form of carbohydrates, circulating in your blood. These glucose molecules came from the carbohydrate-rich foods that you ate recently.

After 20-25 minutes of working out, your body should have already consumed most of the glucose in your blood. The low blood sugar concentration will make it look for other sources of energy. The usual source of energy is the glucose we have stored in our body in the form of glycogen. Many obese people have high amounts of stored glycogen in their bodies. This stored glucose will be converted into usable form and used for your workout.

When much of your glycogen has been converted and used, the body will turn to another energy-source which is our fat reserves. The fats in our body will also be converted into glucose and used up.

If we continue to work out, we will reach a point where the body will already use the protein in our muscles as a source of energy. We don't want to reach this point because protein should only be used as an energy source in emergency situations.

You can't expect to consume all your stored glucose in one workout session. Depending on your weight, it may take months or even years if you only workout 2 times a week. To increase the pace of glycogen reduction, you should make sure to work out regularly and to schedule them effectively.

Your Workout Schedule

In the beginning, when your enthusiasm is up, you should try to get as much workout as possible. If this is your first time working out using the kettlebell exercises, you may get some muscle sore in some muscle groups after a few sessions. It's good to deal with that now while your enthusiasm in working out is still at its peak.

After completing the 30-day kettlebell WoD, you should already see some results. You should not stop your workout habits however. You could continue working out at regular intervals. You could try spreading your workouts all throughout the week if your schedule is crowded for daily workouts.

There are times when you need reduce your workout sessions to 3 or 4 per week. When you spread your workout sessions evenly throughout the week, you will have an increased metabolic rate in most of your waking hours. If you work out 4 times a week for example, you could distribute your sessions on Monday, Wednesday, Friday and Saturday.

The metabolic effects of your workout on Monday will still continue and begin to lessen on Tuesday. By Tuesday evening or Wednesday morning, your metabolic rate will be back to normal.

By working out again in Wednesday morning, you will raise your metabolic rate again and continue its effects on Thursday. This cycle together with the right eating habits, will significantly increase the speed at which you reach your goal.

Chapter 9: Low Carb Diet

For you to lose weight faster, you must accompany your kettlebell regimen with the right type of nutrition. You must achieve balance between not eating too much and not starving yourself. You should remember that your body needs energy so that you can continue working out. People often eat less when they work out because they think that it will yield results faster. The combination of high-intensity workouts and low-calorie intake often ends in disaster.

People who do this type of workout and nutrition regimen easily become tired. They also don't perform well in workout sessions because of the lack of glucose in their systems. When they do workouts that use weights, they often experience hypoglycemia.

There is an easier way to get the results that you want fast. You just have to eat the right types of foods. More specifically, you must make sure that you minimize the amount of carbohydrates in your diet. Carbohydrates are an essential nutrient in maintaining and fueling our bodies. However, because of the abundance of carbohydrate-rich foods, we have become accustomed to consuming more than the prescribed amount of carbohydrates.

It is the main reason why the number of overweight people is increasing year after year. If you are on the heavier side of the scale, you should check your habits if you are consuming too much carbohydrates.

Starting a Low Carb Diet

If you want to start a low-carb diet, you should first learn what to eat and what not to eat. Basically, you want to maximize the protein-rich foods that you take in. It is okay to eat carbohydrates before your workouts. After the workouts however, you should make sure that you minimize breads and grains and focus on meats.

You should also monitor the types of meat that you eat. Minimize your ingestion of red meat and focus more on white meat. Ideally, you should eat a lot of fish. If you are located in an area where fresh fish is scarce or expensive however, you could use poultry as an alternative. Chicken is the cheapest option but you could also checkout other types of poultry or fowls available in your area.

You could also eat red meat but you should not consume it regularly. If you are making a choice between the different types of red meat, choose the ones that feed on grass rather than artificial feeds.

Chapter 10: The Paleo Diet

Paleo diet is highly recommended for people who are trying to start a healthy eating lifestyle. It is a variation of the low-carbohydrate diet. The idea behind Paleo diet is simple; if the food wasn't available to cavemen, then it is not included in your diet. This means that you can only eat the types of meats and plants that did not undergo processing. You can eat grain but you can't eat bread. You can eat roasted meat but you can't eat canned meat. It's easy to make the distinction of what can be and can't be eaten.

By using this diet, you don't have to deal with meticulous thinking of the types of calories that you eat. In some cases, you can even eat until you are full and you will still lose weight and get in shape.

What can I eat?

The Paleo diet creators suggest that since our ancestors were hunters and gatherers back in the days, the majority of our diet should be made up of food that could be obtained through hunting and gathering. Meat is a crucial part of this diet. If you are building muscles and you need to load up on protein, you could add nuts into your diet. We can eat most plant based foods around us as long as we eat them in their natural form. Cave men did not have the technology to preserve their food. That means that we should not eat dried, salted or pickled foods.

Grains are still acceptable but we should eat them in a quantity that also mimics the availability of grains back in prehistoric times. At that time, it is expected that men relied on grain that grew in the wild. They did not farm nor process it. They ate them in their naturally cooked state.

Lastly, you should also take note of the seasonal fruits available in your area. Our ancestors relied on these fruits for vitamins. Some types of fruits will also satiate your craving for sweets. Every time you find yourself craving for a piece of cake, you should grab a piece of mango instead.

How will this affect my energy level during the day?

By limiting the amount of grains and processed foods that you eat, you are limited to only a few options in your diet. The lack of the usual carbohydrate-rich grain will lessen the amount of simple sugar that goes into your system. Most of the sugar that you will take in should occur naturally in nature. They are not as abundant as the glucose we usually take in when we eat bread or rice. They are also not as easily digested and absorbed.

The lack of simple sugar in your diet will prompt your body to look for more glucose and they will focus on the stored carbohydrates in your body. Your body will start converting glycogen into glucose. During workout day, when your body is in need of more energy, it will tap into your fat reserves and convert that into glucose.

If you follow the workout plan in this book together with the Paleo diet, you will have the toned body that you want. To make it less boring, you should learn to mix and match between the meat, peanuts, fruits and the small amount of grains.

Conclusion

Thank you again for purchasing this book on kettlebell workouts!

I am extremely excited to pass this information along to you, and I am so happy that you now have read and can hopefully implement these strategies going forward.

I hope this book was able to help you understand how kettlebell based workouts can help in weight loss and how to apply the basic principles into actions that produce results.

The next step is to get started using this information and to hopefully live a fit, active and happy life!

Please don't be someone who just reads this information and doesn't apply it, the strategies in this book will only benefit you if you use them!

If you know of anyone else that could benefit from the information presented here please inform them of this book.

Finally, if you enjoyed this book and feel it has added value to your life in any way, please take the time to share your thoughts and post a review on Amazon. It'd be greatly appreciated!

Thank you and good luck!

Preview Of:

Ultimate Carb Cycling Guide!

<u>Carb Cycling</u>

Quickly Lose Fat, Preserve Muscle Mass, And Build Self Confidence With Sustainable Fat Loss Carb Cycling Diet Tips And Strategies That Work Fast!

Introduction

I want to thank you and congratulate you for purchasing the book, *Carb Cycling: Ultimate Carb Cycling Guide! - Quickly Lose Fat, Preserve Muscle Mass, And Build Self Confidence With Sustainable Fat Loss Carb Cycling Diet Tips And Strategies That Work Fast!*

This book contains proven steps and strategies on how to plan your own carb cycling diet with explanations of the concept, the science behind it, and several food recommendations.

Have you heard of cyclic ketogenic diet? No? Well, that isn't a bad thing. You probably already know about it, more popularly known as carb cycling.

To keep one's body fit, there are a lot of things to consider. One of those is attaining an ideal weight. If you already have an ideal weight, then it's just a matter of maintaining it. If you're overweight, then you have to reduce weight. If you're underweight, then you should gain weight. But you shouldn't just stop with the numbers you see on the weighing scale. Your body's composition is also important. When losing or gaining weight, you must be sure that you are losing fat and gaining muscle.

Two things play the greatest part here: diet and physical activity. Weight is about the calories: how much you get from the food you eat and how much you spend on the physical things you do. There should be a correct balance between them. Diet and exercise go hand in hand in this matter. Although these two things can be discussed together, our main focus here is dieting.

Thanks again for purchasing this book, I hope you enjoy it!

Chapter 1: Understand The Concept Of Carb Cycling

There have been a lot of diets formulated since long ago. You probably heard of many whether you've been searching or not. To a certain extent, all of them can work since diet is basically calorie deficit. Consume less than what you spend and you lose weight. The thing is that a healthy weight is not just about the quantity but also the quality. It is not just how much you eat that matters, but also the kind of food you eat. Diet can get a little complicated especially if you have further goals such as building and toning your muscles or gaining an ideal body for a specific sport.

Carb cycling is one of the many diets popular among body-builders and athletes. That's because it can build and maintain muscle mass. Also, it adds efficiency in fat burning.

Carb cycling may have its roots from bodybuilding but now it gained significance even in the general health community. That explains a good part of why it's getting a great deal of attention nowadays. Since you're reading this book, it's quite likely that it got your attention, too. You probably want an in-depth learning of carb cycling. So, let's finish up this introduction and get to the good part: learning about carb cycling and how to apply it.

In order to effectively apply carb cycling into your own lifestyle, you must understand deeply its concept. As mentioned earlier, the science behind the diet can get really complicated. But don't worry. You don't really need to go into all the technical terms and whatnot in order to understand carb cycling, or any diet for that matter. This book will still discuss the science behind carb cycling but it can be simplified enough for the average person.

What is carb cycling?

Controlling carbohydrate intake has been of great importance when talking about nutrition. Studies abound regarding the relation of improper carbohydrate intake to serious health concerns such as chronic diseases and obesity. But still, carbohydrates are also important for our body. So, it is not always just about reducing the carbohydrates you consume, but actually taking in the right amount of carbohydrates.

The above is the reason why carb cycling and similar diets were formed. The carb cycling diet uses an approach of alternating the level of carbohydrate consumption. Such a diet involves periods of zero, low and high carbohydrate intake. As it turns out, it isn't just about taking in the right kind and amount of carbohydrates but also taking them at the right time. The kind of carbohydrates, how much, and when you will take them influence how your body responds to them.

In a carb cycling diet, you schedule your week into no-carb, low-carb, and high-carb days. Note that a high-carb day doesn't mean you'll pig out on carbs – you still control the amount but just higher compared to the other days. You'll see more on that later.

A carb cycling diet doesn't only take carbs into consideration. There's also protein and fat – taking the right amount of these is equally important. Throughout the schedule, you need a high level of protein intake. For fat, it is inversely proportional to your carb intake. Thus, during zero or low-carb days, your fat intake should be high. During high-carb days, you consume low fat.

Carb cycling diets will be varied in terms of specific protocols. However, they all share the same basis. The structure is simple: a few days of low-carbs, one day of high-carbs, followed by a day of zero-carbs or low-carbs, and the cycle goes back to the beginning.

As an example, you may schedule four consecutive days of low-carb, high-carb the next day, zero-carb after that, and back to the beginning. Or, schedule three consecutive days of low-carb, one high-carb day, and then back to low-carb.

To gain insight on what is involved in a carb cycling diet, here are some numerical figures:

- On a high-carb day, your set amount of carbohydrate intake is generally between 2 to 2.5 grams for every pound of body weight. Protein intake is set at 1 gram for every pound while fat intake is set to 0 to 0.15 grams for every pound.

- On a moderate-carb day, carbohydrate intake is 1.5 grams for every pound. Protein is at 1 to 1.2 grams for every pound, and fat is at 0.2 grams for every pound.

- On a low-carb day, the intake is at 1.5 grams of carbohydrates for each pound of weight. Protein intake is generally increased to around 1.5 grams per body pound, and fat goes up to 0.35 grams for every pound.

- A zero-carb or no-carb day doesn't really mean zero carbohydrates at all. The term is just for distinguishing from the low-carb since the no-carb day has a really low limit. It no longer takes into consideration body weight – you must not go over 30 grams of carbohydrates for the whole day. Here, you consume 1.5 grams of protein for every pound and fat rises up to 0.5 to 0.8 grams for every pound. Note that this zero/no-carb day is skipped by some people. It is up to your goals or what fits your level of physical activity.

As you can see, the diet involves a detailed measurement of the carbohydrates, protein, and fat that you consume. It takes a lot of discipline especially if you have specific goals. You must really get into the diet if you want to accomplish it. However, once you start, you'll find that it is not as difficult to incorporate to your daily lifestyle compared to other types of diet. Furthermore, this book is a good starting point.

Thanks for Previewing My Exciting Book Entitled:

"Carb Cycling: Ultimate Carb Cycling Guide! Quickly Lose Fat, Preserve Muscle Mass, And Build Self Confidence With Sustainable Fat Loss Carb Cycling Diet Tips And Strategies That Work Fast!"

To purchase this book, simply go to the Amazon Kindle store and simply search:

"CARB CYCLING"

Then just scroll down until you see my book. You will know it is mine because you will see my name "Mia Conrad" underneath the title.

Alternatively, you can visit my author page on Amazon to see this book and other work I have done. Thanks so much, and please don't forget your free bonuses

DON'T LEAVE YET! - CHECK OUT YOUR FREE BONUSES BELOW!

Free Bonus Offer: Get Free Access To The www.LiveFitVIP.com VIP Newsletter!

Once you enter your email address you will immediately get free access to this awesome newsletter!

But wait, right now if you join now for free you will also get free access to the "The 7 Keys To Body Transformation" free EBook!

To claim both your FREE VIP NEWSLETTER MEMBERSHIP and your FREE BONUS Ebook on THE 7 KEYS TO BODY TRANSFORMATION!

Just Go To:

www.liveFitVIP.com